50 DIY Beau~~ty~~ ~~Recipes~~ Using Ev~~eryday~~ Ingredients

Natural, Homemade
Skin, Hair and Body Care

Tara Evans

Just to say "thank you" for buying this book, I'd like to give you a bonus gift

absolutely free

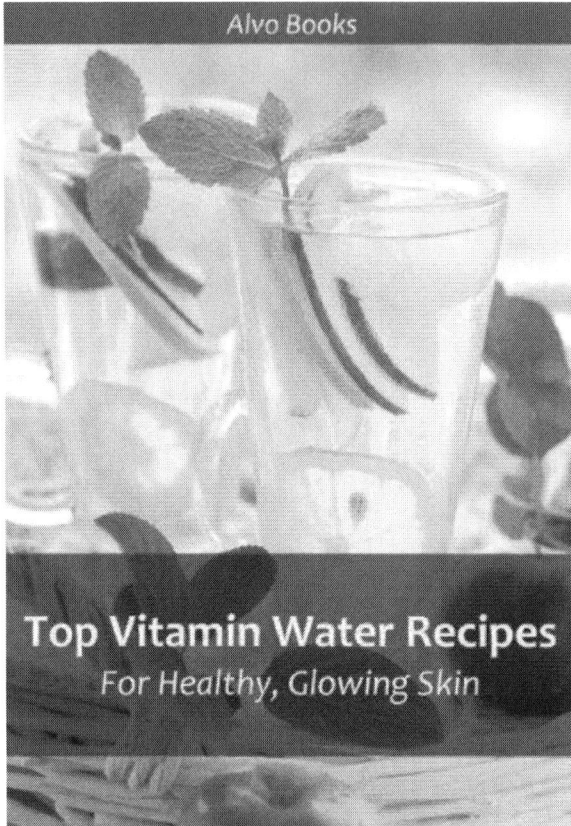

To claim your copy, go to:
www.alvobooks.com/naturalbeauty

Contents

Introduction

If you're looking to pamper yourself but don't want to spend hundreds of dollars at a spa, then this book is for you! I've compiled my favorite quick and easy recipes that you can make from products found in the kitchen. You can treat yourself and not break the bank with these easy homemade beauty recipes. Better still, since the ingredients are all natural, they are free from harsh chemicals and are full of vital nutrients for your skin, hair, nails, and body. Get ready to enjoy the luxurious natural recipes in this book all in the comfort of your own home.

Precautions

As with all new skin care regiments, make sure you test a small area of skin prior to use. Avoid contact with eyes and take care with other sensitive areas. If you notice any recipes or ingredients causing irritation, discontinue use immediately.

Take care with any recipe that uses lemon or carrots as both can cause the skin to be photosensitive. This means they may cause an exaggerated reaction in some people such as sunburn, rash, or blistering. If you know you are going to be in the sun for a prolonged period of time, you might want to consider skipping that recipe for the day or make sure everything has been washed off thoroughly.

Another thing to keep in mind as you switch to more natural and organic products is that there will be a transition phase. For example, you may notice that your skin or hair is producing a little more oil at first as your body rids itself of the chemicals and toxins from synthetic products. Keep at it as your body will find a natural balance after this detox phase settles down.

Basic Ingredients

These recipes are super easy to make and the ingredients are things you already have in your pantry. As I made the transition from store bought skincare to homemade skincare I was so excited to see how many ingredients I already had in my kitchen! I prefer to buy organic products for cooking when I can, which works well for my skincare recipes.

I've included a list of some of the most common ingredients in this book and their benefits for your skin.

1. **Oatmeal** and **black eyed peas**, are exfoliating ingredients you will find throughout the book. These are best used ran through the food processor or blender for a few seconds to grind into smaller pieces. They provide your skin with a gentle, natural exfoliant without causing irritation.

2. **Apple cider vinegar** has numerous uses for your household, but in this book we are focusing on its benefits for your skin and hair. Ideally, you should use raw, unfiltered, organic apple cider vinegar. This means it has retained the top medicinal properties. Apple cider vinegar helps reduce skin inflammation and also helps strip build up on the hair while leaving it soft and shiny! As an extra bonus, it helps reduce dandruff.

3. **Baking soda** cleans the hair without any parabens or sulfates. It is a natural deodorizer and helps absorb excess oil.

4. **Honey** is full of antioxidants for your skin which will help fight wrinkles and signs of aging. It will help clarify your skin and fight blemishes, and cleans your hair. If you consistently use honey on your hair, you may notice some lightening. I usually only use the honey recipes once a week in the winter, and every other week in the summertime when my hair is exposed to more sunshine.

5. **Olive oil** and **coconut oil** are both excellent moisturizing oils that help nourish your skin.

6. **Brown** and **white sugar** are both great for exfoliation.

7. **Ground coffee** is another good source for exfoliation. The caffeine will give your skin an extra 'boost' and it is backed with antioxidants to help fight the appearance of aging skin.

8. **Plain yogurt** will provide your skin with several different vitamins and minerals. The recipes containing yoghurt can help clear acne, reduce the appearance of pores, and lighten the appearance of your skin.

9. **Rose water** increases circulation to the skin while balancing the pH levels. Having a balanced pH level

decreases the chances of skin irritation and acne break outs. You can generally find rosewater at your local supermarket in the skin care section or ethnic ingredients section, or you can visit your local health food/supplement store.

10. **Herbs** such as rosemary, lemongrass, and peppermint leaves add a lovely aroma to the recipe and carry some of the plant's natural benefits.

11. Various **spices** such as ginger and cinnamon help renew the skin, encourage new cell growth, and help combat skin irritations.

Scrubs

The recipes in this section are great for exfoliation and moisturizing. You can package these in mason jars and decorate for handmade gifts your friends and family will love.

Chocolate Sugar Body Scrub

You can never go wrong with chocolate. This chocolate sugar scrub not only smells delicious but will leave your skin smooth and soft! This scrub can be stored in an airtight container for around 4 weeks at room temperature.

Ingredients:
1. 1 cup brown sugar
2. ½ cup cocoa powder
3. ½ cup olive oil
4. 2 teaspoons ground cinnamon
5. 2 tablespoons vanilla extract

Directions:
1. Mix together all ingredients in a large bowl.

2. Place mixture in your chosen airtight container.

3. Gently massage chocolate scrub into skin, avoiding the face.

4. Rinse off thoroughly with warm water.

Cinnamon Oatmeal Scrub

This scrub is great for the entire body. The cinnamon and honey will cleanse the skin while the oatmeal gently exfoliates. This scrub is great for sensitive skin! It will last for about a week if refrigerated or for 2-3 days at room temperature.

Ingredients:
1. 1 cup ground oatmeal
2. 2 tablespoons ground cinnamon
3. 2 tablespoons honey
4. ¼ cup olive oil

Directions:
1. Grind oatmeal in the blender or food processor for a few seconds.

2. Mix in ground cinnamon.

3. Slowly add honey and olive oil.

4. Apply directly to the skin, scrubbing gently before washing off.

Vanilla Almond Scrub

Treat yourself with this luxurious body scrub. It will leave your skin soft and polished all day. This scrub will last about 2 weeks if refrigerated, and 1 week if held in an airtight container unrefrigerated.

Ingredients:
1. ¼ cup almonds
2. ½ cup olive oil
3. 1 cup coarse sea salt
4. 2 teaspoon vanilla extract

Directions:
1. In a blender or food processor, grind almonds into a fine powder.

2. Mix all ingredients together and place in an airtight container.

3. To use, gently rub body scrub into skin.

4. Rinse off thoroughly with warm water.

Soothing Peppermint and Rosemary Salt Scrub

Treat your skin to this calming body scrub! These ingredients will do wonders for your skin and the soothing fragrances from the herbs will help your whole body relax. It will last for several weeks stored at room temperature in an airtight container.

Ingredients:
1. 1 cup coarse sea salt
2. ¼ cup baking soda
3. 3 tablespoons dry peppermint leaves
4. 3 tablespoons dry rosemary leaves
5. ½ cup grape seed oil

Directions:
1. Mix together all ingredients.

2. Gently massage salt scrub into skin.

3. Rinse off thoroughly with warm water.

4. Pat dry.

Java Body Scrub

There's a lot to love about this recipe! Caffeine can be absorbed by the skin and will encourage a more youthful, healthy appearance. This recipe can be stored for several weeks at room temperature in an airtight container.

Ingredients:
1. 1 cup coffee grounds
2. ½ cup brown sugar
3. ½ cup olive oil
4. 2 teaspoons ground nutmeg

Directions:
1. Mix ingredients together in large bowl.

2. Place in your chosen reusable container.

3. Massage a small handful of scrub onto entire body.

4. Rinse off with warm water and pat dry.

Delicious Chocolate Coconut Scrub

As wonderful as chocolate and coconut are for your taste buds, your skin will love them even more! This recipe can be stored at room temperature in an airtight container and should last about a month.

Ingredients:
1. 1 cup brown sugar
2. 2 tablespoons cocoa powder
3. 3 tablespoons finely shredded, dried coconut
4. ½ cup coconut oil
5. ¼ cup olive oil

Directions:
1. Thoroughly combine all ingredients.

2. Store in an airtight container for continued use.

3. Gently scrub the body and let mixture soak into skin for a few minutes (I don't use this on my face).

4. Rinse off thoroughly.

Plumping Lip Scrub

This recipe will gently exfoliate and moisturize your lips. The cinnamon will increase circulation to your lips giving you a plumper and rosier look. This recipe will make enough for a few uses and will last several weeks. Make sure to store at room temperature and in an airtight container.

Ingredients:
1. 1 teaspoon brown sugar
2. 1 teaspoon honey
3. ½ teaspoon ground cinnamon (optional)

Directions:
1. Mix ingredients together.

2. Store in airtight container.

3. Gently massage scrub onto lips and let sit for about 5 minutes.

4. Wipe off with warm wash cloth.

Exfoliating Foot Scrub

Take care of your feet with this wonderful scrub. The Epsom salt and ground split peas will help remove dead skin and the olive oil will leave them feeling silky smooth. If you don't already have Epsom salts in your bathroom cupboard, you can easily find them at your supermarket or drug store. This mixture should be refrigerated between uses, and will last about two weeks.

Ingredients:
1. 1 cup Epsom salt
2. ½ cup olive oil
3. ¼ cup dried split peas
4. 2 teaspoons lemon juice

Directions:
1. Using a food processor or blender, grind dried split peas to a fine consistency.

2. In a large bowl, mix ingredients together thoroughly.

3. Soak feet in warm water for 10 minutes.

4. Then take your time and massage the scrub onto each foot.

5. Rinse off thoroughly and pat dry.

Zingy Citrus Scrub for Legs

Refresh and invigorate your senses and legs with this citrus scrub! This is a great way to exfoliate before shaving. This mixture will last for several weeks stored at room temperature. Keep out of direct sunlight.

Ingredients:
1. ½ cup olive oil
2. 1 cup coarse sea salt
3. ¼ cup lemon juice
4. 2 teaspoons lemon zest
5. 2 teaspoons grated ginger

Directions:
1. Mix all ingredients together in an airtight container.

2. Gently massage scrub onto legs.

3. Rinse off thoroughly with warm water.

4. Pat dry or apply shaving cream.

Gardener's Hand Scrub

Of course the best way to avoid getting dirt under your nails is to wear gloves while gardening. Personally, I can't standing wearing gardening gloves. This usually results in my hands being perpetually dirty throughout the summer. If you're a gardener, or you just want a great cleansing and softening scrub for your hands, this is for you! This recipe will last for several months stored at room temperature. Try to avoid direct sunlight and store in an airtight container.

Ingredients:
1. 1 cup white sugar
2. ¼ cup coconut oil
3. ½ cup citrus liquid dish soap
4. 2 tablespoons lemon zest
5. 1 tablespoon lemon juice
6. 1 tablespoon dried lemongrass

Directions:
1. Mix together all ingredients in a large bowl until completely combined.

2. Put your scrub into your chosen airtight container.

3. Using a small amount of hand scrub, work into hands and forearms for a few minutes before rinsing off with warm water.

4. Pat dry.

Masks

Masks are a great way to revitalize your skin. These recipes will help nourish in many different ways. You can give your skin a wonderful glow with these masks. I would recommend starting out using the masks once or twice a week as they are either very richly moisturizing or very good at exfoliating.

Anti-Aging Face Mask

Papaya naturally exfoliates your skin and is packed with antioxidants to decrease the signs of sunspots and wrinkles. This recipe will make enough for 1-2 uses and can be refrigerated for several days.

Ingredients:
1. 2 tablespoons ground oatmeal
2. 3 tablespoons plain yogurt
3. 1/4 ripe papaya

Directions:
1. Mix together oatmeal and yogurt in a bowl.

2. Slowly mash in papaya, making sure everything is evenly dispersed.

3. Apply mixture generously to the face and neck, allowing it to sit for 10 minutes.

4. Using warm water, wipe off face mask with wash cloth and pat dry.

Rejuvenating Banana Face Mask

Give your skin a healthy boost of nutrients from bananas, while the lemon juice and honey help to clarify your skin. This recipe will make enough for 1 application and is best made when you're ready to use.

Ingredients:
1. ½ plain yogurt
2. ½ slightly overripe banana
3. 2 teaspoons honey
4. ½ teaspoon lemon juice

Directions:
1. Mash banana and yogurt together in small bowl.

2. Mix in honey and lemon juice.

3. Apply mask generously to the face, allowing mixture to sit for 10 minutes.

4. Wash off thoroughly with warm water.

Chocolate, Raspberry, and Yogurt Face Mask

This scrumptious mask will lightly moisturize and help fight breakouts. The raspberries act as a natural astringent for your skin. This recipe will make enough for 1 mask application. If you wish to make a larger amount, it will store in the refrigerator for about 1 week.

Ingredients:
1. ½ cup raspberries
2. ¼ cup plain yogurt
3. 1 teaspoon cocoa powder
4. ¼ cup ground oatmeal

Directions:
1. Mash raspberries in a bowl.

2. Mix in cocoa powder, oatmeal, and yogurt.

3. Apply mask generously to face and neck and let sit for 10-15 minutes.

4. Gently wipe off with warm wash cloth.

Scar Refining Mask

If you have ever dealt with acne in your life then you have probably experienced some sort of acne scarring. I battled with hormonal acne in my teens and went through a series of microdermabrasion treatments to remove the scars that were left behind. This process was painful and left my skin red and flaky for several days after each session. Instead, this mask helps reduce the signs of scarring and is much gentler on the skin! This recipe makes enough for 1 application. It can be stored in the refrigerator for up to a week.

Ingredients:
1. ½ cup oatmeal
2. 4 drops lemon juice
3. ½ teaspoon ground cinnamon
4. ¾ cup water

Directions:
1. Add water and oatmeal to a microwave safe container.

2. Microwave for 1 minute or until oatmeal is cooked well.

3. Mix together cinnamon and lemon juice well.

4. Allow paste to cool for a few minutes before applying to face.

5. Let paste sit for 15-20 minutes before wiping off with a warm damp wash cloth.

6. Cover face with cool damp towel for 5 minutes.

7. Repeat this mask once every 2 weeks over a 6 week period, followed by once a month applications if needed.

Moisturizing Avocado Face Mask

This mask is super versatile for the whole body. You can use it everywhere from your face to dry elbows and even your feet! Your skin will be left feeling silky smooth. This makes enough for 1-2 applications and should be stored in the refrigerator between uses. If you choose to store it, the avocado will discolor.

Ingredients:
1. 1 ripe avocado
2. 2 tablespoons olive oil
3. ¼ cup ground oatmeal
4. 1 tablespoon honey

Directions:
1. Peel and remove seed from avocado and mash it.

2. Grind oatmeal in food processor or blender.

3. Mix all ingredients together.

4. Apply mask to desired areas and allow it to dry for 10-15 minutes.

5. Wipe off gently with warm wash cloth.

Rise and Shine Face Mask

Awaken your skin with a caffeine boost! The ingredients work together to fight blemishes and reduce the signs of wrinkles. This recipe will make enough for 1 mask but if there is extra, make sure it's stored in an airtight container in the refrigerator.

Ingredients:
1. 2 tablespoons ground coffee
2. 2 tablespoons plain yogurt
3. 1 tablespoon honey
4. A pinch or two of ground cinnamon

Directions:
1. Mix all ingredients together in small bowl.

2. Apply directly to face and neck.

3. Let mask sit for 10 minutes and wash off with warm water.

Moisturizing Papaya and Avocado Foot Mask

Papaya and avocado are both wonderful moisturizers for dry, cracked feet. This mask will exfoliate dead skin cells on your feet while repairing damaged areas. This recipe makes enough for one application and can be stored in the refrigerator for 2-3 days.

Ingredients:
1. 1 avocado (a slightly overripe avocado works best)
2. ¼ ripe papaya
3. ¼ cup honey
4. ¼ cup plain yogurt

Directions:
1. Mash avocado and papaya together in small bowl.

2. Add in honey and yogurt.

3. Apply mask generously to both feet, focusing on troubled areas.

4. After 10-15 minutes, wash off with warm water.

Watermelon Mask for Sunburns

The watermelon will help repair your skin with its vitamin A and C, while the coconut oil and honey work to moisturize. This recipe makes enough for 1 application.

Ingredients:
1. ¼ cup watermelon
2. 2 tablespoons honey
3. 1 teaspoon coconut oil

Directions:
1. In a small bowl, mash watermelon to a pulp.

2. Add in honey and coconut oil, mixing thoroughly.

3. Apply mask to sunburned area and allow to sit for 20 minutes.

4. With cool wash cloth, gently wipe off mask.

Cooling Body Mask

Great for after sun care or long hot summer days. This mask should be stored in the refrigerator between uses and will last for about a week.

Ingredients:
1. 1 bag chamomile tea
2. 1 medium sized cucumber
3. ½ cup aloe vera gel (fresh from your garden, or gel from your bathroom cupboard is fine too)

Directions:
1. Brew large mug of chamomile tea.

2. While mug is cooling, puree cucumber in blender.

3. Mix together aloe vera, cucumber puree, and tea.

4. Apply mask to body, letting it cool for 15-20 minutes.

5. Wash off thoroughly.

Bath Time

Every now and then it's great to take a little personal time! I've compiled some of my favorite relaxing bath recipes for you to enjoy as well. I would recommend grabbing a good book and a nice drink and let yourself be pampered.

Spicy Coconut Milk Bath

Treat yourself to this delicious bath and let your skin soak up all of the benefits that come from the coconut. You can store the dry ingredients together for several months, and when you're ready to use, simply add in the coconut milk.

Ingredients:
1. 2 cups coconut milk
2. ½ cup coconut oil
3. 1 cup finely shredded dried coconut
4. 2 tablespoons ground cinnamon

Directions:
1. Mix together all dry ingredients in an airtight container.

2. Draw a warm bath.

3. When you're ready for your bath, mix in ½ to 1 cup of the dry mixture and 2 cups of coconut milk.

4. Soak for 20-30 minutes.

5. Pat dry.

Rosemary Peppermint Bath

A refreshing and invigorating bath that will leave you feeling relaxed! This mix can be stored for several months in an airtight container at room temperature.

Ingredients:
1. 2 tea bags of peppermint tea
2. 1 cup coarse sea salt
3. 2 cups Epsom salt
4. ¼ cup dried rosemary
5. ¼ cup dried peppermint leaves

Directions:
1. Mix all ingredients together in an airtight container (except the tea bags).

2. When you're ready for your bath, draw a warm tub of water.

3. Add in your two bags of peppermint tea and ½ to 1 cup of your bath mixture.

4. Soak for 20-30 minutes.

5. Pat dry.

Rose Milk Bath

Treat your skin to this ultimately nourishing and rejuvenating bath! This mixture could be stored for several months at room temperature without the rose water.

Ingredients:
1. 3 cups powdered milk
2. 2 cups rose water
3. ½ cup coconut oil
4. 2 cups coarse sea salt

Directions:
1. Mix together all ingredients except rose water in an airtight container.

2. When you're ready for your bath, draw a tub of warm water.

3. Pour in ½ – 1 cup of bath mixture and add the rose water.

4. Soak for 20-30 minutes.

5. Pat dry.

Chamomile and Calendula Bath

This bath is great if you feel like you need to regenerate. The chamomile and calendula help to renew and repair your skin. You can store this mixture in an airtight container for several months.

Ingredients:
1. 1 cup loose leaf chamomile
2. 1 cup loose leaf calendula
3. 2 cups Epsom salt

Directions:
1. Mix all ingredients together in an airtight container.

2. Draw a warm bath.

3. Pour in ½ to 1 cup of chamomile bath mixture.

4. Soak for 20-30 minutes.

5. Pat dry.

Soothing Bath Mixture

This bath mix is wonderful after too much time in the sun. This recipe makes enough for one bath but if you do store it, refrigerate for up to a week.

Ingredients:
1. 1 cup Epsom salt
2. 1 cup apple cider vinegar
3. 3 bags green tea
4. 3 teaspoons ground ginger

Directions:
1. Draw a warm bath.

2. Add in ingredients and mix well.

3. Soak for 20-30 minutes.

4. Pat dry.

Detoxifying Sea Salt Bath

Help relax sore muscles with this soothing bath salt mixture. Epsom and sea salt is great for increasing blood flow and helps detoxify the body. This mixture can be stored for several months in an airtight container at room temperature.

Ingredients:
1. 2 cups Epson salt
2. 1 cup coarse sea salt
3. 1 cup rose water

Directions:
1. Mix all ingredients together in your chosen container.

2. When ready, draw a warm bath.

3. Add in ½ – 1 cup of mixture.

4. Soak for 20 – 30 minutes.

5. Pat dry.

Hair Care

Most of us suffer from one type of hair damage or another. Whether your hair has dried out from too much heat with styling or color treatments, there are several recipes in this section to help tame your hair and give it natural shine once again!

Moisturizing Hair Serum

This serum is great to help repair dry, or chemical or heat damaged hair. The oils will help repair split ends and the honey will help lock in moisture. This serum can be stored for 3-4 weeks at room temperature in an airtight container

Ingredients:
1. ½ cup olive oil
2. ¼ cup coconut oil
3. ¼ cup honey

Directions:
1. Mix all ingredients together.

2. Apply generously to ends, working your way up to your scalp.

3. Tie hair loosely in a bun and let serum sit for 1 hour, or overnight. (If you sleep with serum in, make sure your put a towel down to protect your bedding.)

4. Wash out thoroughly in the shower with warm water.

Anti-Dandruff Scalp Scrub

This scrub will help you beat dandruff and will encourage healthy hair growth. This scrub can be stored in an airtight container at room temperature for about 1 week, or for 2-3 weeks in the refrigerator.

Ingredients:
1. ½ cup brown sugar
2. ¼ cup olive oil
3. 2 teaspoons honey
4. ½ cup apple cider vinegar
5. 2 teaspoons grated ginger

Directions:
1. Mix all ingredients together.

2. Apply thoroughly to wet hair.

3. Massage scrub into scalp and roots.

4. Rinse out completely with warm water.

5. Use as needed once a week.

Shampoo Substitute with Baking Soda

If you're looking for a hair care method free from synthetic ingredients, the best way is to avoid using traditional shampoo and conditioner. Baking soda isn't a detergent, so it won't dry up the natural oils on your hair and scalp. It will help by absorbing extra oil and removing dirt. The cinnamon in this recipe helps encourage hair growth. I wouldn't recommend storing this recipe.

Ingredients:
1. 1/4 cup baking soda (possibly less depending on your hair type)
2. 1 cup water
3. 1 teaspoon ground cinnamon

Directions:
1. Mix water and baking soda together in a cup. Baking soda should be thoroughly dissolved before use.

2. Carefully apply mixture to roots and scalp, massaging gently. There is no need to apply mixture to the full length of the hair as the main goal of this shampoo is to absorb any excess oil.

3. Make sure you rinse baking soda out thoroughly before following with the apple cider vinegar rinse in the next recipe.

4. You may need to adjust the amount of baking soda you use as time goes by depending on the amount of oil your scalp produces.

Conditioner Substitute with Apple Cider Vinegar

This will add shine to your hair while removing build up from synthetic products. It will also help detangle your hair and add a lovely shine. As your hair dries, it will soften and smooth out. Don't worry! The smell of the vinegar goes away as your hair dries.

Ingredients:
1. 1 cup apple cider vinegar
2. 1 cup water

Directions:
1. Mix water and vinegar together.

2. Work into hair and scalp, massaging gently.

3. Rinse thoroughly.

Strengthening Hair Mask

Great for brittle, heat damaged hair. Give your locks an extra boost of strength with this mask! Make sure you don't rinse out with hot water, as the egg will cook on your hair. This recipe needs to be used soon after making it – I wouldn't recommend storing it.

Ingredients:
1. 2 eggs
2. ½ cup olive oil
3. 2 teaspoons grated ginger

Directions:
1. Crack two eggs into a bowl.

2. Whisk in olive oil and grated ginger.

3. Apply generously to wet or dry hair and let set for 10-15 minutes.

4. Using cool or lukewarm water, thoroughly rinse out mask.

5. Shampoo and condition like usual after.

Deep Conditioning Avocado Hair Mask

This recipe is a great fix for dry, damaged, and color treated hair to give it back a healthy shine. This recipe makes enough for one hair mask treatment and can be repeated weekly if needed. It's best made when you're ready to use it as the avocado will discolor if stored.

Ingredients:
1. 1 ripe avocado
2. ½ cup olive oil
3. 1 teaspoon lemon juice
4. 2 tablespoons apple cider vinegar

Directions:
1. Peel avocado and remove seed.

2. Mash and mix all ingredients together.

3. Apply mask evenly to hair and work gently into scalp.

4. Allow mask to sit for 30 minutes – 1 hour.

5. Wash out thoroughly in the shower.

Dry Shampoo for Light Hair

For those days when you are running behind and don't have time to wash your hair, dry shampoo is a great time saver. Your dry shampoo can be stored for several months in an airtight container at room temperature.

Ingredients:
1. ½ cup cornstarch
2. ½ cup baking soda
3. Old foundation makeup brush to use for application.

Directions:
1. Mix baking soda and cornstarch together in an airtight container.

2. To apply, gently dab brush into mixture and tap off extra powder.

3. Take small section of hair around the crown of your head and brush in small amount of dry shampoo.

4. Repeat, applying small amount of powder to the roots along the crown of your head.

5. Allow powder to sit and soak up extra oils for a few minutes before brushing out any excess.

Dry Shampoo for Dark Hair

This dry shampoo recipe is better for darker hair but can be used the exact same way as dry shampoo for light colored hair. Your dry shampoo can be stored for several months in an airtight container at room temperature.

Ingredients:
1. ½ cup cornstarch
2. ½ cup baking soda
3. 3 tablespoons cocoa powder
4. Old foundation makeup brush to use for application.

Directions:
1. Mix baking soda, cocoa powder, and cornstarch together in your container.

2. To apply, gently dab brush into mixture and tap off extra powder.

3. Take small section of hair around the crown of your head and brush in small amount of dry shampoo.

4. Repeat, applying small amount of powder to the roots along the crown of your head.

5. Allow powder to sit and soak up extra oils for a few minutes before brushing out any excess.

Herbal Rinse for Light Hair

This recipe is for those of you with lighter hair colors that are looking for a moisturizing rinse for your locks without any additives that will turn your hair a dark, dingy color over time. If desired, you can add in a few drops of lemon to gradually brighten your hair. This recipe will last for about a week if stored in an airtight container at room temperature or two weeks refrigerated.

Ingredients:
1. 1 cup of freshly brewed chamomile tea
2. 1 cup apple cider vinegar
3. 1 cup water
4. Reusable container (I use a squirt water bottle with a sealable cap on the top)

Directions:
1. Mix together all ingredients in your chosen container.

2. Apply rinse to wet hair and work in well with your hands.

3. Let rinse sit for 10 minutes before rinsing out well with warm water.

4. Shake container well before each use.

Herbal Rinse for Dark Hair

For anyone who has dark hair, this recipe is great! Give your hair an extra boost of strength and shine. This recipe will last for about a week if stored in an airtight container at room temperature or two weeks refrigerated.

Ingredients:
1. 1 cup freshly brewed black tea
2. 1 cup apple cider vinegar
3. 1 cup water
4. Reusable container (I use a squirt water bottle with a sealable cap on the top)

Directions:
1. Mix together all ingredients in your chosen container.

2. Apply rinse to wet hair and work in well with your hands.

3. Let rinse sit for 10 minutes before rinsing out well with warm water.

4. Shake container well before each use.

Sea Salt Hair Spray

This recipe is an easy way to get beautiful beach hair and natural waves. You can add texture to your hair and style afterwards, or let your hair air dry and enjoy natural waves. This spray can be stored at room temperature in a spray bottle for several months.

Ingredients:
1. 1 tablespoon hair gel
2. 2 tablespoons coarse sea salt
3. 1 tablespoon olive oil
4. 1 cup water
5. 1 teaspoon lemon juice (optional)

Directions:
1. Mix together all ingredients in a spray bottle. The lemon juice will add a little extra texture and can be used to gradually lighten your hair over time.

2. Shake spray bottle well between each use.

3. Spray generously on hair and scrunch gently.

Makeup Routine

This section is dedicated to natural alternatives for some of your makeup routine. When you're turning over to a more natural and holistic skincare regimen, it's easy to forget that your store bought makeup and remover can be packed with harsh chemicals. I have included some of my favorite homemade alternatives you can include in your daily routine.

Eye Makeup Remover

A super-easy way to remove your eye makeup. It is very gentle and moisturizing on the skin.

Ingredients:
1. 1 tablespoon olive oil
2. Clean wash cloth

Directions:
1. Pour olive oil onto hands and gently rub onto eyes, paying close attention to eyelashes.

2. Take wash cloth and soak in warm water, then wring out extra water.

3. Set wash cloth on the face until it cools.

4. Wipe off residual oil and makeup with wash cloth.

Silky Makeup Remover Wipes

These wipes are perfect for removing makeup all over the face and neck without leaving your skin feeling too oily, or getting makeup all over your bath towels. This recipe will normally last for 3-4 weeks at room temperature.

What you need:
1. 1 roll strong paper towels
2. 1 very sharp knife
3. 2 cups warm water (preferably water that was boiled and then allowed to cool to a warm temperature)
4. 3 tablespoons coconut oil
5. Reusable airtight plastic container.

Directions:
1. With the sharp knife, carefully cut paper towel roll in half and set aside extra half of roll.

2. Remove inner cardboard tube from paper towel roll.

3. Drop coconut oil and warm water into your chosen plastic container and mix until coconut oil is completely melted.

4. Place the half of paper towel roll you are working with into your plastic container and allow roll to absorb the water and coconut oil mixture.

5. Once roll is fully wet, you can squish down the roll until it fits into your container and close the lid.

6. To use, open container and remove 1-2 sheets of your new wipes and gently remove your makeup!

Berry Lip Stain

A great way to add beautiful color to your lips! Refrigerated, this will last for a week in an airtight container.

Ingredients:
1. 1 blackberry
2. 3 red raspberries
3. ½ teaspoon coconut oil

Directions:
1. Mash blackberry and raspberries together, squeezing juices into your chosen container.

2. In a microwave safe container, melt coconut oil with 10 second intervals.

3. Add in melted coconut oil and mix well.

4. Allow lip stain to cool and harden before use, then simply apply to your lips.

Beet Red Lip Stain

If you're looking to add a little more color to your life, beet lip stain is the way to go. It will be a little more dramatic than the previous lip stain recipe and will literally stain everything, so take care when making this recipe! This recipe can be stored in the refrigerator for 1-2 weeks in an airtight container.

Ingredients:
1. 1 large beet
2. 2 drops lemon juice (helps preserve color)
3. 1 tablespoon coconut oil

Directions:
1. Blend beet well in a blender or juicer. Squeeze out as much juice as possible into a separate container.

2. In a microwave safe container, melt coconut oil in microwave in 10 second intervals.

3. Mix together lemon juice, melted coconut oil, and beet juice into your chosen container.

4. Allow lip stain to cool and harden. To use, apply directly to your lips!

Homemade Bronzing Powder

Give yourself a natural summer glow all year long with your own homemade bronzing powder. Because everyone has a different skin tone, you'll need to play around with the ratio of ingredients to get your desired shade and tone that works best for you. I have quite fair skin naturally, but I do get out in the sun quite a bit, so the amounts in this recipe work for my very slightly tanned skin tone. This recipe can be stored for several months in an airtight container at room temperature.

Ingredients:
1. 2 tablespoons cornstarch
2. 1 teaspoon ground cinnamon
3. 1 teaspoon cocoa powder
4. 1 teaspoon ground nutmeg

Directions:
1. Mix together your ingredients adding more nutmeg and cocoa powder for a darker shade, and cinnamon for more of a reddish tone. Cornstarch will help you lighten your bronzer if you accidentally go too dark.

2. Put your bronzer in your chosen airtight container.

3. Use as you would any other bronzer and avoid contact with the eyes.

Extras

This section has several different options that you can incorporate into your regular skin care routine. I use these recipes in my weekly skin care routine and I absolutely love them!

Pore Cleansing Gelatin Strips

For this recipe, you can definitely use plain gelatin which generally seems to be a little less expensive, but from personal experience, I try to stick with a scented gelatin. I struggled with the scent of plain gelatin, but didn't have any issues with the flavored variety. Use whatever works best for you! If you choose to use a flavored gelatin, make sure you stick to neutral colors (peach was the closest to my skin tone). If you pick any bold colors, they will leach out onto your face and will make a mess everywhere!

Ingredients:
1. 1 packet of peach gelatin (or plain gelatin)
2. 1-2 tablespoons of water

Directions:
1. Mix peach gelatin together with water in a microwave safe container

2. Warm mixture in microwave for 5-7 seconds. Watch carefully, as mixture can bubble over quickly and unexpectedly.

3. Gelatin solidifies quickly so apply 'goo' onto problem areas avoiding eyes and any other sensitive spots.

4. Allow mask to sit for 15 minutes, or until all areas are thoroughly dry.

5. Peel off mask and enjoy your smooth skin!

Gentle Facial Toner

Using a facial toner in your daily skincare routine is important. After cleansing the skin, the natural pH balance is typically thrown off. A facial toner helps to bring your skin back to its regular levels and prevent blemishes from forming. This particular facial toner is good for all skin types, but is especially great for sensitive skin.

Ingredients:
1. Rose water
2. Reusable plastic spray bottle

Directions:
1. Fill spray bottle with rose water.

2. Cleanse face and neck like normal.

3. Lightly spray rose water onto skin and neck area.

4. Allow to air dry then follow with your normal moisturizer.

Blemish Fighting Toner

This toner is for all skin types and focuses on fighting and preventing blemishes. The mixture will last for several weeks stored in an airtight container at room temperature.

Ingredients:
1. 1 bag green tea
2. 1 mug of boiling water
3. 2 tablespoons apple cider vinegar
4. ½ cup filtered water
5. Spray bottle

Directions:
1. Brew 1 mug of green tea and let cool.

2. Mix all ingredients together in spray bottle.

3. To use, cleanse face as normal.

4. Shake spray bottle well before each use.

5. Spray generously onto face and let air dry.

6. Follow with your usual moisturizer.

Eye Brightening Treatment

Reduce the appearance of dark circles naturally with this easy recipe! For best results, use this treatment weekly and make sure you are consistently getting an adequate amount of sleep each night.

Ingredients:
1. 1 small pealed potato
2. 1 mug freshly brewed green tea
3. 1 teaspoon coconut oil

Directions:
1. Brew 1 cup of green tea, and let cool

2. Slice the potato into small round sections.

3. Let two slices of potatoes soak in green tea for 10 minutes.

4. Place potato rounds over your eyes and sit back to relax for 20 minutes.

5. Remove potatoes and gently wipe off any excess liquid on the skin.

6. Gently dab a small amount of coconut oil under eyes to moisturize.

Refreshing Lime Foot Soak

Relieve your aching feet with this refreshing mint and lime foot soak. The Epsom salts with help relieve soreness while the lime and peppermint will leave them feeling and smelling fresh. This recipe can be stored in an airtight container at room temperature for several months. If you plan on storing your soak for later use, make the recipe without the lime juice and then add it directly into your warm water.

Ingredients:
1. 1 tub of very warm water
2. 1 lime
3. 2 teaspoons lime zest
4. ¼ cup dried peppermint
5. 1 cup Epsom salt
6. ¼ cup baking soda

Directions:
1. Mix all dry ingredients together, including the lime zest.

2. When ready to use foot bath, squeeze in lime juice and add 3-4 tablespoons of dry mix into warm water.

3. Let feet soak for 10-15 minutes.

4. Pat dry.

Rehab for Nails

I struggle all year round with dry, brittle nails that never get the chance to grow. One of the best things I've done for my nails is this treatment! They're much stronger and I don't have to worry about them breaking during daily activities. You can store this nail treatment in an airtight container at room temperature for several months. I use this on my nails and hands nightly before bed.

Ingredients:
1. 2 tablespoons coconut oil
2. 1 teaspoon olive oil

Directions:
1. Mix both ingredients together and store in an airtight container.

2. Rub well onto nails, cuticles, and hands.

3. Works well for an overnight foot treatment too!

Nail Strengthening Soak

Soak your nails once or twice weekly to give them an extra boost of nutrients and help protect them.

Ingredients:
1. ½ cup rose water
2. 2 teaspoons honey
3. ¼ cup milk

Directions:
1. Mix ingredients together thoroughly in a shallow bowl.

2. Let nails soak for 10 minutes.

3. Shake off extra water and let air dry.

4. Follow up with a moisturizer.

Spot-on Pimple Treatment

Whenever you notice a pimple starting to form, wipe it out with this natural spot treatment! This treatment can be stored at room temperature in an airtight container for 2 weeks.

Ingredients:
1. 1 tablespoon of honey
2. 1 teaspoon of ground cinnamon
3. 1 drop lemon juice

Directions:
1. Mix together all ingredients until they form a paste.

2. Apply treatment to breakout area and let sit for 10-15 minutes.

3. Gently rinse and wipe off with warm water.

4. Pat dry.

Silky Smooth Leg Shaving Cream

Never buy an over the counter shaving cream again! This recipe is very moisturizing for your legs and helps give you a smooth, even shave. This recipe can be stored at room temperature for about a month in an airtight container.

Ingredients:
1. ¾ cup shea butter
2. ¾ cup coconut oil
3. 2 ½ tablespoons baking soda
4. ½ cup olive oil
5. 2 teaspoons lemon juice

Directions:
1. In a microwave safe container, melt coconut oil using 10 second increments.

2. Add in all other ingredients except baking soda, mixing thoroughly.

3. Let mixture set for a minute or two to cool.

4. Add in baking soda and mix thoroughly until it resembles a cream or frosting.

5. Apply to legs when ready to shave.

Conclusion

Now that you've had a chance to try the recipes in this book, you'll realize that it's quick and easy to make your own beauty treatments at home. It's also a lot of fun and actually cheaper than buying conventional products. Best of all, you know that your treating your skin, hair, and body with all natural ingredients that are free from toxins and are completely safe for you, your family, and the environment.

Can I Ask You a Favor?

I'm so glad you enjoyed this book enough to make it all the way to the end and I hope you've found it really useful. If you liked the book, would you be open to leaving an honest review? That would really help out other people who are looking for a book on the topic and it also helps us as a small, independent publisher.

To leave a review, simply go to the relevant Amazon page in your country.

Thank you!

15783697R00040

Printed in Great Britain
by Amazon